Contents

Introduction

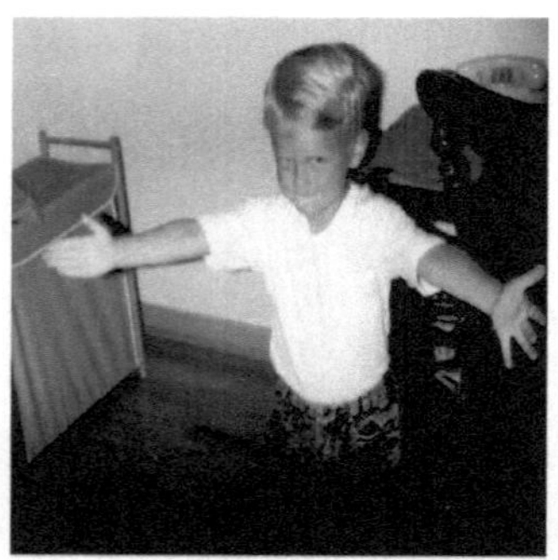

Me at age five.

I am writing this book because I hate seeing people, especially children, suffer from unnecessary health problems. My struggle with asthma from a young age is very personal to me as I remember the emotional trauma vividly. The feeling of not being able to breathe as a young child is a scary experience. Heck, it is scary even for adults.

A quick disclaimer, I am not a licensed doctor, nor do I pretend to be one. The FDA makes people like me say this because they have cornered the market on "proper healthcare", even though their methods did nothing for my well-being long-term or for the treatment of my condition. Please discuss everything you read in this book with your doctor before implementing.

I do believe more medical doctors are coming around to alternative medicine, but it is hard to do so when most medical textbooks are written or endorsed by pharma companies. It's hard to make good decisions with bad information. The best piece of advice ever given to me was "follow the money". If you can successfully connect the dots by following the money, you can draw your own conclusion as to whether the information presented is in your best interest or a profiting third party's best interest.

Lastly, as a child, do you remember all the playtime of pretend? For example, let's pretend to play "house" or "firemen/police". As we grow into adults, we seem to forget the power of playing pretend. I personally healed my asthma by playing "doctor". Even in the health care industry, they still call it practicing medicine. Don't be afraid to listen to your own body for guidance on how to heal. Shoving pills into your mouth isn't always the answer to your health problems. Our bodies are wonderfully designed like an exotic supercar but think about the problems caused if given the wrong type of fuel. Can you imagine pouring olive oil or rubbing alcohol into the gas tank of a Lamborghini? Sadly, we think nothing of doing something similar to our very own bodies, and we wonder why our bodies break down on us over time.

I am not one for writing fluff, and it is my desire to get straight to the answers, but I want to shape the conversation so you have a solid understanding about the approach I took; not solely looking for an immediate quick fix. I'm trying to get your mindset away from aerosol inhalers and into a lifestyle that promotes whole body health and healing. This is not only important for adults to understand but adults who have children that suffer from asthma as I did. Most children will not understand the shift in diet, and might feel left out from their peers, so it is the job of the parent to be the role model, teacher, and source of encouragement. If you truly love yourself or your child, you will do things that may not always be popular, easy, or convenient.

In the upcoming chapter, I give my personal account of my experience suffering from asthma from age five until age sixteen. I've written this part, so you may identify the stage you might find yourself. Due to a lack of knowledge, my parents made many errors when handling my case of asthma. The Internet back then was not how it was today, and unfortunately, they relied on the doctors to help in this matter. However, we never got to the root cause of my asthma, and the doctors only temporarily masked the symptoms with prescription drugs. I will share my background from the time I was an infant and show you where things began to take a turn for the worse with my health. Looking back as an adult, I can now pinpoint the cause and effect in relation to my asthma. It is my sincere hope that my experience will bring you relief and ultimate healing without further pharmaceutical dependency or possible long-term lung damage.

Peak Flows, Sleepless Nights, And Pale Face

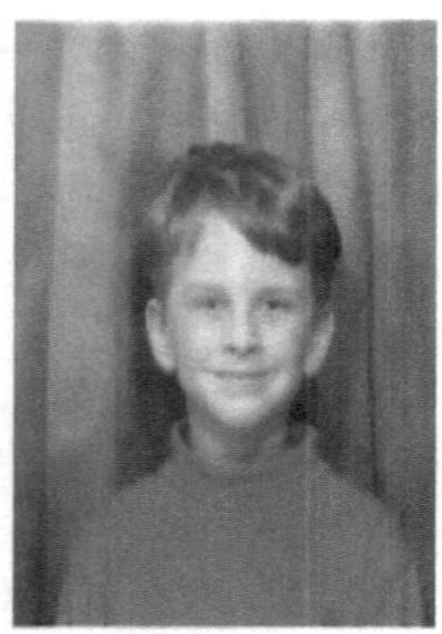

Me at age eight.

The title of this chapter sums up my early childhood experience to the tee. My early life revolved around having my peak flows taken and written down, my Albuterol inhaler in my cargo pocket at all times, and a face that was usually on the pale side.

A good night's rest was a luxury at times, especially when I had a cold, or spring, summer, and fall allergies were making my symptoms worse. My father and I used to joke about my pale face due to my shallow breathing which would now be considered politically incorrect. As I sat in the kitchen puffing on my nebulizer he would say, "How, pale face?" And I would say back between puffs, "How! Me not so good." It was the best my father and mother could do as I'm sure they felt helpless. Asthma was my sole experience. No one else in my family could feel what I was feeling. Looking back at myself, I didn't realize how brave of a child I was. Laying in my bed at night, I would quietly listen to the symphony of little wheezes and crackles coming from my small chest and lungs. It eventually became the norm for me.

I was born on August 25, 1985, an only child. I received five doses of DTP, four doses of Polio vaccine, and two doses of MMR. It was shortly after July of 1990 at age five that I began to display minor Tourette's. Unfortunately, this is something that has stayed with me my entire life. Also, on August 25,1986, I presented with transient erythroblastopenia. My asthma began to present roughly around age five-and-a-half, and I was formally diagnosed in April of 1991. My medical records can be seen on the next pages.

IMMUNIZATION RECORD

STATE OF WISCONSIN

NOTE: [fine print, illegible]

JONATHAN (MATTHEW)
FIRST NAME

WICHMANN
LAST NAME

8 25 85
BIRTHDATE

IMMUNIZATION	DOSE 1	DOSE 2	DOSE 3	DOSE 4	DOSE 5
DTP	10 24 85	1 7 86	5 27 86	4 8 87	7 11 90
POLIO	12 24 85	1 7 86	4 8 87	7 11 90	
MEASLES	12 16 86				
RUBELLA	12 16 86				
MUMPS	12 16 86	7-11-90 mmR			
Td					

SOCIAL SECURITY NUMBER — ZIP CODE OF BIRTHPLACE: 5 3 3 / 6

SUGGESTED IMMUNIZATION SCHEDULE

1st YEAR OF LIFE	2nd YEAR OF LIFE			SCHOOL ENTRY	REPEAT ANY TIME OF LIFE
DTP POLIO	MEASLES RUBELLA	MUMPS DTP	POLIO	DTP POLIO	Td BOOSTERS

PHYSICIAN OR HEALTH DEPARTMENT PROVIDING IMMUNIZATION

NAME: Dr. Wilton P. Milwl, Wis. PHONE 414 445-6995
NAME: D.R. Johnson PHONE 771-8228
NAME: Dr. Agoncillo PHONE (   )

ADDITIONAL IMMUNIZATIONS	TYPE OF IMMUNIZATION	DATE	TYPE OF IMMUNIZATION	DATE

SPECIAL HEALTH PROBLEMS

My Childhood Eating Patterns

Strangely enough, I distinctly remember easy access to my refrigerator and pantry that was filled with poison masquerading as "food". To give you an idea of what I had access to, I've written a bullet list below:

- Pringles Potato Chips

- Lays Potato Chips

- Different types of sugar cereals like French toast, Captain Crunch, Fruit Loops, etc.

- Spaghettios

- Hostess treats.

- Processed cheese and dairy products.

- High fructose and nasty filler elements in products like Fruit Gushers, Oreos, etc.

As I consider all those products available on the grocery store shelf, it's a shame so many people, including my parents, believed these items were good for human consumption. Also, during this period, the concept of organic had not caught on in the Midwest. It was not clear as to what things were organic or not. This included milk, cheese, meats, and fruits and veggies. GMO corn was rampant and placed in just about everything. My childhood meals consisted of grilled cheese sandwiches, hot dogs, milk, salty snacks, crackers, and sugary treats. High amounts of the wrong type of sodium was present in everything I consumed during those early years.

My Childhood Yearly Medical Routines

Our doctor recommended yearly flu shots as he believed it would help protect me from asthma attacks. Back then, I was allergic to almost everything; mold, dust, and dampness—you name it, and it probably impacted me. I remember feeling sad because I loved animals, but I could have either limited to no contact with them as that would cause my asthma to flare up. My life was fairly isolated and sterile due to the fear that something might trigger my asthma. We had limited to no carpet in the house, my mom was OCD about dusting, and if one of my friends even had a hint of a cold, we could not play together on that day. Asthma brought about a life of isolation and fear.

My doctor ordered allergy shots to help with my problem, and I remember going weekly to get them. That lasted for about a year. I cannot begin to tell you how much of my early childhood life was spent in hospitals and doctor offices. During the "flu" season each year, I was easily rushed to the urgent care center three to five times when my normal medicine didn't stop my asthma attacks. To complicate matters, there is a direct correlation between proper breathing patterns and panic attacks. Since I was young, there were times when I could not determine the difference between an asthma attack and a panic attack. Each one felt the same, and the symptoms I experienced were similar.

Adding insult to injury, when I still got the flu even after getting my flu shot, it would last for weeks because my immune system was suppressed. I remember being prescribed many rounds of amoxicillin and can still remember the taste to this day. If this is beginning to sound depressing and hopeless, that's because it was, and that was my life for quite some time. When did things begin to change? When things got even worse for my family.

The Beginning Of My Healing

At the age of fourteen, my mother was diagnosed with breast cancer. Because the term cancer carried so much weight, it felt like a death sentence to us all. I believe this news was even scarier since we lost my uncle to leukemia a few years prior to my mom's diagnosis. I could remember how he looked, and I translated that image to what would eventually happen to my mother. Life began to move fast after the news of my mom's cancer. The doctors pressured her into having a mastectomy, but she did refuse chemotherapy afterward when she read a book written by Dr. Lorraine Day.

I don't remember the exact protocol that was given in the book, but I do remember our entire lifestyle changing rapidly. All the garbage food could no longer be found within our house. Everything we ate as a family was raw and organic. The Outpost, which is like Whole Foods before Whole Foods was prevalent in the Midwest, was the only place we shopped for groceries. We had a daily routine of juicing carrots and dark, leafy greens.

An example of what we juiced is shown below:

- Kale

- Chard

- Spinach

- Broccoli

- Cabbage

- Celery

- Green Apples

- Ginger

- Beets

I remember our family would buy a twenty-five-pound bag of carrots each week. Dr. Day's book might have mentioned the Gerson therapy because looking back on the juicing protocols, they closely reflected what I've read of

Gerson in my adult years. The doctors told my mom that anyone who didn't submit to chemotherapy usually lasted about five years afterward. Nineteen years later, my mom is still alive and cancer-free.

During that initial year of radically changing our lifestyle, I noticed my asthma symptoms and inhaler dependency disappearing. At age fourteen, I was enrolled into a nearby martial arts program where I learned proper deep breathing exercises. My American Sifu knew a few things about eastern medicine and pointed me toward a new path that I knew nothing about. It was the best thing that had ever happened to me as it brought me to where I am today. By age sixteen, I was completely free from asthma.

To put everything into perspective, here is a list of things I took and/or couldn't do:

- Intermittent usage of prednisone.

    -Stunting of growth

- Daily usage of Albuterol inhalers.

    -This had a side-effect of making me hyper or giving me the jitters.

- Albuterol nebulizer in-home treatments.

- Yearly Flu shots.

- Allergy Shots.

- Allergic to pollen, dogs, cats, hay, and much more.

- Many rounds of antibiotics.

- Very light exercise. I could not run even a quarter mile.

All the items above went away within one year of our family lifestyle and diet change. Now that you're familiar with my personal story, let's get into the actual protocol that I believe will help you heal asthma in the same way mine was healed.

Whole Body Approach

Eastern medicine knows that the entire body works together as one, and nothing is ever isolated. Western "treatments" usually always target the immediate problem at hand. Example: You can't breathe, so you take a puff on your inhaler. The solution inside your inhaler is designed to target any inflammation or irritation inside the lungs. However, they don't take time to figure out why the body is producing inflammation, or why the human immune system is in a constant state of weakness.

Based on my personal experience with asthma, if I had to sum the main causes, I would assign blame to inflammation and poor gut health. By changing our lifestyles back when I was fourteen, we corrected these two things, but I never knew why. Fast-forward to present time, I not only know the "why", I understand how it all works together. Let's explore the steps required to begin healing from asthma.

The Asthma Protocol

One thing I would immediately have done is a comprehensive IgG food sensitivity test. This can make you aware of certain foods that are having a high inflammatory response within the body. Once you know what those food sensitivities are, cut them from your diet. When you have asthma, all dairy products must go. No milk, cheese, butter, or yogurt. Only after you have healed from asthma should you consider reintroducing dairy in very small amounts. Because I have gone for so long without dairy, I don't care to eat it. Also, because of the severity of my asthma, and the length of time I suffered, this was a small sacrifice for me to make.

Do your best to switch over to all organic produce and products. Your diet should consist of minimal to no processed foods. Basically, if it's in a box, avoid it. Raw, whole foods need to become plentiful in your daily diet. All white sugar must be removed from your diet. This includes sweets, sodas, and yes, especially diet sodas! Also, greatly reduce sodium/salt intake during your healing process.

Begin to look at the labels on everything you buy. If you can't pronounce something or wouldn't find it in nature, avoid it. Bread, wheat, and pasta products also need to be removed. You want to avoid creating a glue-like substance within your gut. During this time, we will be working on restoring the health of your gut and ultimately your immune system. We want to starve the body of refined sugars, bleached flour, starches, artificial anything, and mucus creators like dairy. Caffeine or similar stimulates must also be removed.

I have found a modified version of the keto diet is ideal for people suffering from asthma. I am not suggesting eating high animal content like meat and chicken, but rather a higher fat diet from plant-based sources. An example of this would be avocados and certain nuts and seeds. This diet can be a better alternative because it starves the body of processed sugars and flour-based products. This leads me to the next section: gut restoration.

Gut Protocol

This part is extremely important for both adults and children. Almost everyone has been exposed to a round of antibiotics, eaten garbage food for years, fast food, and high sugar. All these things play a part in deteriorating the health of your gut. Our bodies are amazing as they can adapt over time to any changes we are making, whether good or bad.

When we feed our body high amounts of sugar, the bacteria that cultivates in our gut produces more of the little guys that are meant to process sugars. However, over time, an overgrowth of the wrong types of bacteria remain in your gut and begin to take over. This can lead to all types of imbalances and problems. One thing that personally helped me as I worked to heal my gut was the adoption of a mono diet for a few weeks. Here was my step-by-step approach:

1. Take the food sensitivity test and view results.

2. Remove and stay away from my highest triggered food types that were on my report.

3. Pick foods that are in my lowest categories, and only eat those for two weeks. An example would be fresh, raw beans, salad lettuce, and avocados (I didn't eat any fruit during this time; only a banana in my morning smoothie).

4. Right when I wake up before I eat or drink anything, I take an ounce of aloe vera juice. The brand I like is shown below. You do not need to take this forever, just for a week or two.

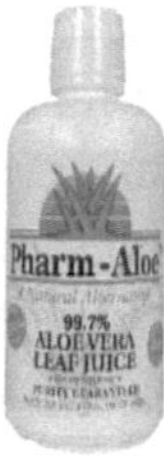

1. Take a soil-based probiotic. The two brands I like and mix together are shown below. These I take daily right when I wake up.

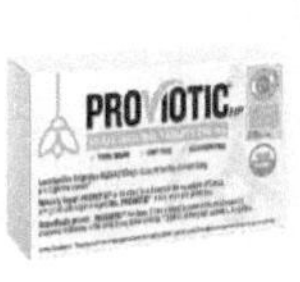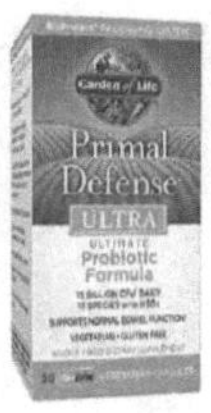

2. After thirty minutes to an hour has passed, I make my morning smoothie to break my fast. Here are the ingredients I put into my NutriBullet blender:

3. One medium-sized banana, one scoop of Carrington farms organic coconut and pea protein blend, a teaspoon of Hodgson Mill Flax and Chia blend, one scoop of Dr. Axe Multi-Collagen Protein, a generous helping of frozen blueberries, one tablespoon of organic peanut butter, and lastly, a quarter teaspoon of NOW brand spirulina powder. I drink/eat this over a period of thirty minutes.

4. Throughout the day I will eat as much of my allowed food as needed when hungry. When you have asthma, pure filtered water is your friend. I have been drinking filtered water from a ProPur filtering system ever since I was ten years old. It gets all those nasty, harmful things out, including the poison fluoride.

5. Lastly, I stop eating all food around 6:30 pm at night and only allow myself water. This is called intermittent fasting, and it allows your body to focus on healing rather than long-term digestion. Remember this little saying, "Energy in, energy out." In other words, whatever you put in your mouth should give you a greater energetic return. Every time you put something into your mouth, ask yourself a few of these questions:

a. Does this help my cells rebuild stronger or weaker?

b. Will this cause more inflammation inside my body or less?

c. Will this make me tired, foggy, irritable, or create stomach issues?

You may be asking yourself, "So how long does it take before I begin to see results?" Everyone is different and every body is at a different stage. Because of how bad off I was, it took me six months before I noticed any radical differences with my asthma. Granted, I was super strict with myself during that time, no cheating at all.

Extra Things You Can Do If You Wish

There are a few extra things I recommend if you can afford to add them to your routine. As you switch away from the standard crap American diet, your body will begin to detox. Depending on how much medication you've pumped through your body, and for how many years, your lymphatic system is probably sluggish. The lymphatic system is responsible for cleaning you out. It is the route your body uses to remove harmful cells, regenerate the immune system, keep you virus free, and much more. If the lymphatic system can't keep up with the toxin dump, then the overflow of this drainage system empties into the bloodstream without complete filtration.

Here are a few things you can do to keep that lymphatic system moving:

- Go for a lymphatic massage. Yes, it's a real thing.

- Buy a rebounder trampoline and jump on it for about 12–15 minutes a day.

- Work out! Flexing muscles act like a pump and move the fluid as well.

- Drink the recommended amount of water per day.

- Take a hot/cold shower. Basically, this means you stand in the shower with hot water for a minute, then turn it to cold water for a minute. Alternate like this 5-8 times.

In the next chapter, we will discuss how to wean ourselves off our inhalers.

Inhaler Alternative

Have you ever had a panic attack? Do you suffer from anxiety? I would say many people with severe asthma most likely have lingering anxiety and random panic attacks. Many things can trigger a panic attack such as stress, lack of sleep, and remaining on the mental hamster wheel. I've had plenty myself, and they seem to come out of nowhere. These anxiety issues stem from our shallow breathing patterns subconsciously taught to our body through years of suffering asthma.

I remember back when I was a child, I would purposely breathe more shallowly because it hurt when a coughing spasm occurred. Sometimes I was just tired, and it was easier to breathe shallowly. Over time, this became a pattern that followed me into adulthood. This unnatural breathing pattern began to create a "fight or flight" response as my brain was being tricked into thinking something bad was about to happen to me.

Looking back now, I believe 30% of my "asthma attacks" were actually panic attacks that felt like asthma attacks. This led me to develop an almost unbreakable, codependent bond between me and my inhaler.

How do we begin to move away from the dependency of inhalers? I've had great success with diffusing essential oils. I have played around with different blends that work best for having the same impact on the lungs as an inhaler does. The brand I chose to diffuse is Young Living oils. The diffuser I recommend is called TheraPro. I've included a picture of the product below.

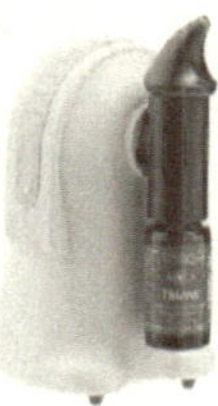

I like this diffuser because of how small the particles are diffused. I list the blends of what I diffuse below, but I want to clarify when/how to use this diffuser. In my opinion, prevention of any disease, including asthma, is the best method, not intervention. I don't recommend turning to the diffuser during a full-blown asthma attack. In that situation you will need your nebulizer or inhaler, depending on the severity. However, as your body responds to your new diet, and maybe you feel the beginning of a possible asthma attack coming on, go to the diffuser before the inhaler.

The diffuser is great for adults and children because you can pre-diffuse the oil blend in the room before bedtime. The TheraPro has an intermittent on/off timer so you can have it diffuse every twenty minutes for a minute or two all throughout the night. Below are the essential oils you will need to create the blends.

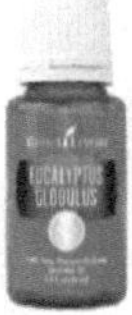

I use Eucalyptus as the base for all my solutions that I inhale through the diffuser. Typically, Eucalyptus will make up 50% of the total solution.

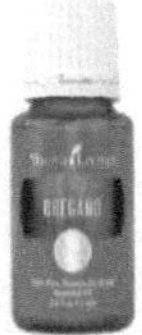

This stuff is super potent but very effective. Oregano makes up about 20% of the solution. Be careful not to get any on your fingers/hands or accidentally touch around your eyes as it can burn.

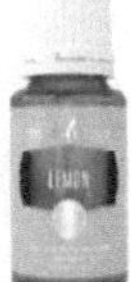

The last 30% of the solution will contain lemon or orange. Lemon is my personal preference. You will then mix all three of these oils into the extra bottle that should come with the TheraPro, using the percentage ratio of 50/20/30.

Turn on the TheraPro diffuser to the midway point and breathe the essential oil mix in deeply through the mouth from about one inch from the nozzle. I would cycle in and out three deep breaths, then turn it off. I would do this a few times throughout the day whether I felt an asthma attack coming on or not.

Oregano has anti-inflammatory properties, and the eucalyptus helps with respiratory relief and is soothing. The lemon works in conjunction with oregano in fighting any potential bacteria or viral infections. The key to healing asthma is to not allow your lungs to become burdened by any outside attacks. We want to keep the stress off the lungs so they can focus on the normal function of breathing, proper oxygen saturation, and the healing of lung tissue and small passageways.

Advance Remedies

I'm including these advanced methods toward the end of this guide because I don't want you, the reader, to immediately rush to buy "health solutions". You must do the work through diet and lifestyle change first. Usually, this is powerful enough to begin the healing process. Every now and then you might need an extra boost, and this is where these extra remedies come into play.

There are two very powerful things you can take, but I recommend you go very slowly as these methods can detox the body too quickly. Also, if you are on any other prescription drugs, you will want to discuss the following with your doctor to make sure there won't be any interference or negative reactions.

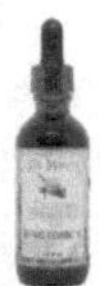

I have used this herbal blend called, Lung Tonic, developed by Dr. Robert Morse. I have found it powerful at clearing the lungs. The ingredient list found in this tincture is as follows:

- Mullein Leaf

- Fenugreek Seed

- Marshmallow Root

- Slippery Elm Bark

- Chickweed Herb

- Bayberry Root

- Comfrey Leaf

- Horehound Herb

- Yerba Santa Leaf

I weigh about 163lbs, and I have found that 1/4 of the dropper is plenty for me. Certain herbs can raise or lower blood pressure, thin blood, and do other things that may interfere with medication or your condition. It is important to not only speak with your doctor, but it is worth the money to have an initial consultation with Robert as well. You can learn more about him and his full line of products on his website.
https://www.drmorsesherbalhealthclub.com

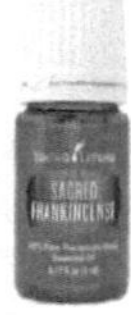

The last little gem within this advanced section is Sacred Frankincense from Young Living. Please note, any essential oil that is ingestible absolutely must say 100% Pure or Therapeutic Grade. Anything else could contain "perfume oil" which is synthetic. This oil can also be added to the TheraPro for inhalation. The compounds found within Frankincense have been discovered to have strong anti-inflammatory and potentially anti-cancer effects.

I would mix a drop or two with a carrier oil like coconut oil and rub it over the chest and lung regions before bedtime. You can also add a drop of lavender to this mix as it has a calming effect and can provide a deep restful sleep to both adults and children. Because of how potent Frankincense is, I would only use it once every other day or third day.

I have personally used Frankincense to help heal a stomach ulcer by either placing a drop in eight ounces of water or in a capsule. **With any essential oil, first apply a test drop on wrist or arm to test for any adverse allergic reaction.** When it comes to children and Frankincense, I would only add a drop or two for diffusing during the night or apply it to the chest as a massage oil as described above. Do not ingest it.

Daily Diet

To encourage the body to heal, I would recommend adhering to this type of diet. I would encourage you to be consistent and refrain from quitting as this way is the proper way humans should be eating anyway.

Juicing is a powerful way to deliver high amounts of nutrition to your cells while allowing your digestion process to rest, reserving all energy for healing. The Kuvings whole juicer is one of the best on the market. You must only use organic produce when juicing, and stay away from high sugar combinations. Things you should be juicing is anything green like celery, cucumber, a handful of cilantro, chard, green apple—like granny smith—etc.

Spinach, I've found, is easier to blend as you don't waste as much product. I recommend doing a juice fast/cleanse once a month. The protocol involves three green juices for one whole day with no food. As you come out of the juice fast into the second day, I would incorporate smoothies and then go back to whole food.

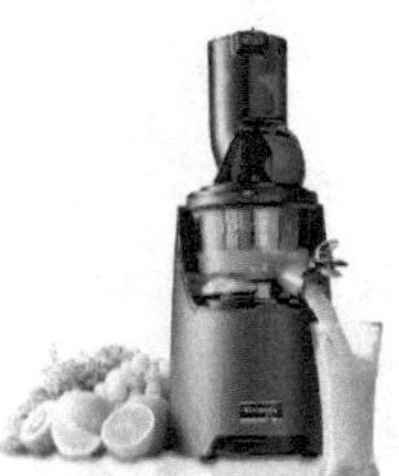

As you are working on restoring gut health, I would recommend not over-combining foods during meals. Keep it very simple. Prepare an organic green salad with fresh toppings like cut up cucumber, carrots, green apple, and tomatoes. Be aware of your IgG report and what you should not be eating. Most vegetables should be reporting in at low levels so it's not a problem. For example: The highest offenders for me are almonds, every part of an egg, cheddar cheese, and cashews.

When it comes to protein, keep it to one handful portion of organic, grass-fed beef or chicken. It is imperative to eat organic meat that has not been shot up with antibiotics or growth hormones as this is passed right along to you through the flesh. This is one reason why I believe most Americans' guts are compromised. The antibiotics they are either consuming or directly taking from doctors does a number on the healthy bacteria within the gut.

When it comes to good and healthy fats, things like avocados, coconut oil, and fatty fish are good. The only caution I would give directly relates to fish. I would only eat fish caught on the Atlantic side or way up north by Alaska. Farm-fed fish is iffy as well because of improper filtration of waste.

After the 2011 nuclear disaster in Fukushima Japan, most of the Pacific Ocean is contaminated, and the sea life is heavily radiated. It's been seven years, and the plant is still spilling radioactive by-product into the ocean and sadly will continue for years to come.

Lastly, supplementing a high-quality spirulina powder into your smoothie is going to be very beneficial.

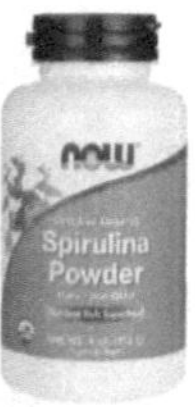

Spirulina is well balanced in crucial vitamins, especially vitamin B. Most people do not absorb or get any benefit from multi-vitamins, and I personally do not recommend them as they are garbage. However, if you can get vitamins from a whole food source, then your body knows how to utilize it better. I have found my workouts are so much better now that I've religiously added this to my morning smoothie.

Spirulina, combined with blueberries, is a one-two knock-out for oxidation that can harm DNA and cells. This type of damage drives up chronic inflammation. Spirulina has been shown to improve symptoms of allergic rhinitis—inflammation in the nasal airways. This nasal inflammation is triggered by environmental allergens like pollen, animal hair, etc. Overall, this is my secret weapon, and I suggest you use it as well.

Exercise For Asthmatics

I remember early on, my mom sheltered me from vigorous exercise because of how easily my asthma was triggered. I don't blame her for doing this because being a parent to a child who suffers from asthma is not easy. I can imagine a parent tends to error on the side of caution. However, I was a persistent and stubborn child and wanted to play sports.

One of the early organized sports I played was soccer. I know, it's a terrible first choice for an asthmatic, but that's what I wanted to do. The coach knew my condition, and I could sub out any time I wanted. I typically played for about five minutes before subbing out. I didn't care because during those five minutes I was as competitive as possible. Eventually, I discovered martial arts and fell in love.

I highly recommend martial arts for children with asthma. If you can find a more traditional "dojo" school, it is better because breathing techniques are taught along with good form. For example: how to exhale when striking, or proper diaphragmatic during cool down and meditation time. In my martial arts school, we were taught Judo as well. This was an interesting sport to participate in as an asthmatic because of the heavy uniform we wore and the close wrestling contact and near smothering that happens.

I think because my mind was active in trying to beat my opponent, I didn't have time to focus on what would have been a prime setup for a panic attack. When you roll around with a partner in Judo, you are typically hot and sweating, your uniform can feel claustrophobic, and some moves can actually smother your face for long periods of time. Doing this type of activity gave me time to learn the difference between a true asthma attack and a panic attack brought on by stressful situations.

Why is this important? Because it stops you from always running to your inhaler when any signs of trouble approach. The less dependent you are on your inhaler, the more time your body has to heal and learn how to cope without medical intervention. As I grew into my pre-teen years, I became more comfortable and knew my limits. I could sit and breathe heavily for thirty minutes until the symptoms began to settle down. As I worked on my diet at age fifteen, my triggers for dust went away. The time frame for runny noses, itchy, red eyes, and sneezing began to taper off until it rarely happened anymore. This was a big sign to me that my body's immune system was functioning properly again and getting stronger every day.

Lastly, I believe swimming is another great form of exercise for those who suffer from asthma. It teaches you how to pace your breathing as your body performs work to either keep you afloat or to swim from point A to point B. When you do the breaststroke, the rhythm forms a good breathing pattern. You are forced to hold your breath as you swim underwater, and you have to create enough force to surface, get a deep breath, and repeat the process again.

Also, while your face is underwater, you breathe out forcefully against the water, essentially doing what you would do with a peak flow monitor. Strengthening your lungs by inhaling deeply and exhaling forcefully, is one key to helping asthmatics. I can't tell you how many years' worth of bad breathing habits I had to overcome because, subconsciously, I was afraid of the coughing and the pain.